Low Carb Cookbook
Delicious Low Carb Diet Recipes

JASON THAWNE

<u>TERMS & CONDITIONS</u>

TABLE OF CONTENTS

Chapter 1 – Delicious Low Carb Diet Recipes

This book is for Low Carb diet recipes. Filled with delicious recipes this is the book you need. Try out these awesome recipes and have a fantastic and delicious breakfast, lunch and dinner!!

Supreme Cauliflower with Sujuk Sausages

This recipe is awesome as well as super delightful. I bet you'll love it.

What you need

- One/two-one onion, shredded
- Eight-nine oz. sujuk sausages sliced (or may be red pastrami)
- 2-3 tbsp. olive oil
- One-two teaspoon. Cajun seasoning
- Four cups frozen cauliflower
- 1 green pepper, chopped
- Two-three tbsp. minced garlic

How to prepare

1. Assemble all the items at one place.
2. In a frying pan, sauté onion with olive oil for seven minutes.
3. Squeeze the liquid from shredded cauliflower and combine it to the pan. Sauté the cauliflower with onion for 8 minutes.
4. Now comes the last step.
5. Add in Cajun seasoning and blend. Now you should add in chopped sujuk sausages or pastrami and green peppers.
6. Toss and cook for approximately five minutes. Shift to the plates.

7. Smell the aroma & now you can serve.

Serve: Four-six

Overall Time: Twenty two minutes

Super Cheesy Bacon and Chive Omelet

Ingredients

- Eggs (two, large)
- Cheddar cheese (1-two oz.)
- Chives (two-3 stalks)
- Bacon (2 pieces, cooked)
- Bacon fat (1-two tsp)
- Salt
- Black pepper

How to prepare

1. Crush eggs together and then you should add pepper and salt to taste. Chop chives and shred cheese.
2. Heat skillet and cooking bacon fat until hot.

3. Combine eggs to pot and top with chives.
4. Now please cook until the edges start to set & then add bacon and start cooking for 32 seconds.
5. One thing remains to be done now.
6. Add cheese and use spatula to fold in half. Press to seal and toss above.
7. Warm and serve immediately.

Serves: One-two

AMAZING EGG AND TURKEY SAUSAGE MUFFINS

What you need:

- ½-one teaspoon. salt
- ¼ cup finely shredded onion
- Half-one teaspoon. pepper
- ¼ cup 2% milk
- Six-seven medium eggs
- Eight-9 oz. turkey sausage
- ¼ cup green finely shredded pepper

Instructions:

1. Assemble all items.
2. Preheat oven to 353 °F.

3. Now please gently apply cooking spray to bottom of muffin pan.
4. Cook sausage and then cut in small bites and fill muffin pan half way.
5. Now comes the most important part.
6. Now please mix together: cream, green pepper & eggs and place on top of the sausage.
7. One thing remains to be done now.
8. Please put in the oven & then bake for 22 minutes till fully cooked. Cook till eggs are golden brown.
9. Once done, withdraw and cool for a couple of minutes

before gently spooning every muffin out of the pan. Sprinkle with fresh parsley and/or may be dill.

10.   Smell the aroma and then you can serve.

Makes- Six-seven serves

Preparation time: Twelve minutes

Cooking time: Twenty two minutes

Fantastic Pancakes and Syrup

Sizzle your taste buds and get the taste of this simple yet really tantalizing recipe.

What you need

For pancakes:

- Coconut milk (One/three cup)
- Erythritol (2-3 tbsps)
- Cinnamon powder (One-two tsp)
- Eggs (Four, large)
- Nut butter of your choice (Three/four cup)
- Baking soda (One/two-one tsp)
- Ghee (Two-three tbsps)

For Syrup:

- Sukrin Fiber Syrup
  (One/two cup)
- Maple extract (Two-three
  tablespoons, sugar-free)

Directions

1. Assemble all items.
2. Combine items for syrup to
   a jar and use spoon to stir
   till it is blended thoroughly.
   Cover jar and put apart till
   needed.
3. Put eggs, nut butter,
   erythritol, baking soda,
   coconut milk and cinnamon
   powder in a food processor
   and pulse till blended.
4. Heat ghee in a non-stick
   skillet and then you should
   add batter to pot, use

approximately ¼ cup per pancake. Cook until pancake sets in, then flip and finish cooking. Put on a plate.
5. One thing remains to be done now.
6. Repeat with remaining batter and plate.
7. Sprinkle with syrup and then you can serve.
8. Enjoy!!

Serves: Five-six

MYSTICAL BROCCOLI QUICHE

It is one of the rarest recipes. Chefs all around the world would kill me, if they knew that I told you this recipe. Please don't tell it to anyone.

What you need:

- ¼-1 teaspoon. cayenne pepper
- 1 half shredded low-calorie cheese (light feta)
- 3 cups broccoli
- One-two tsp. ground black pepper
- Six-seven large eggs
- ¼-1 teaspoon. cayenne pepper
- One-two tsp. sea salt

Instructions:

1. Assemble all items.
2. Pre-heat oven to 376°
3. Steam the broccoli but do not overcook.
4. Now we may proceed to the subsequent most important step.
5. Steam the broccoli on the bottom of a nine" pie pan.
6. Top with shredded cheese.
7. Blend: eggs, milk, black pepper, cayenne pepper and sea salt and then stir together.
8. One thing remains to be done now.
9. Now please pour the mixture over the broccoli & cheese.

10.   Bake for thirty two minutes or until eggs are well cooked.
11.   Enjoy!!

Servings: Six-seven

Prep time: Twelve minutes

Cooking Time: 32 minutes

Yummy Anaheim pepper Gruyere Waffles

Have a perfect start of the day with this recipe. You are surely gonna love this.

What you need

- One-two teaspoon. Metamucil powder
- Three-four eggs
- Salt and pepper to taste
- One-two small Anaheim pepper
- One-two tablespoon. coconut flour
- One/four cup cream cheese
- One-two teaspoon. baking powder
- One/four cup Gruyere cheese

Directions

1. Assemble all items.
2. Now in a blender or mixer, please blend together all the ingredients except for the cheese & Anaheim pepper.
3. Once the ingredients are mixed well, combine cheese and pepper. Blend well till entire items are mixed well.
4. One thing remains to be done now.
5. Heaten up your waffle iron. Then pour on the waffle blend and cook for 7 minutes.
6. Now serve hot.

Servings: Two-three

Overall Time: Eighteen minutes

Superb Chicharrones con Huevos (Pork Rind & Eggs)

Ingredients

- Tomato (1, shredded)
- Pork Rinds (one.5 oz.)
- Black pepper
- Onion (1/4, shredded)
- Salt
- Bacon (four-five pieces)
- Eggs (5)
- Avocado (one-2, cubed)
- Jalapeno pepper (2-3 seeds removed and sliced)
- Cilantro (1/4 cup, shredded)

How to prepare

1. Assemble entire ingredients at one place.

2. Heaten up skillet and cook bacon until slightly crisp. Remove from pot and place apart on paper towels.

3. Now you should add pork rinds to pot along with onion, tomatoes and pepper. Keep cooking for 6 minutes till onions are soft and clear.

4. One thing remains to be done now.

5. You should add cilantro, stir together lightly and combine eggs. Scramble eggs and then combine avocado and fold.

6. Smell the aroma and serve.

Serves: Three-four

HISTORIC CHICKEN AND EGG SOUP

What you need:

- Two-three cups cooked spaghetti squash
- 9 cups chicken broth
- Salt and pepper
- Four-five cups chicken, cooked and shredded
- 1 lemon, juiced
- 3 eggs
- ½ bunch fresh parsley

Method of preparation:

1. Assemble entire items at one place.
2. Now you should add the chicken and the broth to

a large pot. Then bring to a boil.

3. Stir eggs and lemon juice together in a different bowl.

4. One thing remains to be done now.

5. Slowly pour the eggs within the chicken broth.

6. Now you should add the spaghetti squash and sprinkle with parsley.

7. Smell the aroma and then you can serve.

Serves: Eight-nine

Preparation time: Twenty two minutes

Cooking time: Twelve minutes

FANTASTIC CHEESE CRACKERS & HAM

This is one of my best recipes. You are surely gonna love this one.

What you need:

- Two-three tablespoons sugar free orange marmalade
- 2-3 tablespoons sesame seeds
- 2-3 oz. deli ham
- Two-three tbsps Sriracha
- One- ½ cups Parmesan cheese, grated
- Eight-nine oz. chive and onion cream cheese spread

- 2-3 tablespoons basil

Directions:

1. Assemble entire ingredients at one place.
2. Make the crackers: put foil or parchment paper on a baking sheet and spray with cooking spray. Using a circular cookie cutter, press the cheese into the cookie cutter then sprinkle with sesame seeds. Bake at 376 degrees for 9 minutes.
3. One more thing remains to be done now.

4. Blend cream cheese, Sriracha and orange marmalade together.
5. When the crackers are done, top with the cream cheese/marmalade now spread and a slice of ham.
6. Enjoy your day!!

Servings: 6-7

Preparation time: Twelve minutes

Cooking time: Nine minutes

TASTY BUTTER-CINNAMON CRISPIES

For everybody who misses cinnamon graham crackers, cinnamon rolls—cinnamon something. This is for them!!

Ingredients:

- Three tablespoons (forty 5 g) butter
- Two to three tablespoons (30 to forty 5 g) powdered erythritol* 1/4 teaspoon ground cinnamon
- Three One/two ounces (a hundred g) plain pork rinds or skins

Different Sweeteners

- Two to three tbsps (3 to 4.5 g) Splenda
- Two to three tbsps (six to 9 g) Stevia within the Uncooked

How to prepare

1. Preheat oven to 352°F (a 180°C, or may be gas mark 4). While it's heating, put the butter in a roasting pan and place it within the oven to soften.
2. In a small dish, mix powdered erythritol and cinnamon.
3. When the butter is melted, dump the pork

rinds within the pan, and toss until they're entirely and evenly coated with butter—this takes a little bit of persistence.

4. Sprinkle the erythritol-cinnamon combination above the pork rinds, stirring the all time, in order to get it as evenly distributed as attainable.

5. Please slide the pan into oven, & then cook it for 6 minutes.

6. Pull it out & whisk once more.

Extra ordinary Omelet

This recipe is not hard on your pocket. So enjoy!!

What you need

- One-two tbsp low-fat cheese, grated
- Salt and pepper to taste
- Two-three tbsp onion, diced
- 2 eggs
- Two-three tbsp bell pepper, diced
- One-two tablespoon skim milk

- One-two tablespoon flour

Let's cook:

1. Assemble all items.
2. Crack the eggs directly into the mug and beat with a fork
3. Now comes the most important steps.
4. Combine the onions and bell peppers, and flour, add cheese, milk, stir till well mixed
5. Top with salt and pepper to taste
6. Place within microwave and

cooking for three
minutes
7. Now serve

Preparation Time-Three mins

Cooking Time-4 minutes

Serving Size-1-2

Legendary Basil Noodles

What you need

- Half cup carrot, diced
- Two-three tablespoons lime juice
- ¼ cup lemon grass, sliced
- 15 shrimps, peeled and deveined
- 1 cup serrano chili peppers, shredded
- ½ cup cherry tomatoes
- One-two tsp salt
- ½ onion

- Two-three tablespoons coconut oil
- Two-three tbsps molasses
- ¼ cup green beans, sliced
- Two basil leaves
- Ten cloves garlic
- ½ cup coconut milk
- 8 cherry tomatoes, halved
- Three cups spiralized zucchini noodles

How to prepare

1. Assemble entire items at one place.

2. Process together salt, lime juice, molasses, garlic, peppers, onion, and half cup cherry tomatoes until smooth.

3. In a greased wok, simmer this mixture, basil, lemon grass for twelve minutes while stirring occasionally. Withdraw lemon grass and basil leaves. Set sauce away.

4. In another pan simmer coconut milk, combine shrimp, carrot, beans and cook for 2 minutes. Add the sauce, mix well

and cook for 4
minutes.

5. Now you should add
zucchini noodles to
the sauce and then
blend well and cook
for 6 minutes.

6. Now serve and enjoy!

Tasty Chocolate Cookie Squares

What you need:

For Crust

- Dark chocolate chips (1-2 cup)
- Cashews (one cup), soaked overnight
- Agave syrup (2-three tbsp)
- Almonds (one cup)

For Topping

- One pinch salt
- Cocoa powder (½ cup)
- Raw honey (¼ cup)

- Coconut oil (one-two cup)
- Coconut cream (¼ cup)

Instructions:

1. Gather all items.
2. Take a small baking pan lined with plastic wrap.
3. Blend almonds, cashews, agave syrup and chocolate chips together and pour into the baking pan.
4. Set aside.
5. Blend coconut oil, cocoa powder, raw honey, salt and coconut cream together and then pour it over crust mixture.

6. Please chill in refrigerator for about two hours or so & then cut within squares while serving.

Powerful Chicken, Spinach, Blueberries & Avocado Salad

What you need

- One cup spinach
- 1/2-1 avocado
- One/four cup blueberries
- One-two cup cubed grilled chicken
- <u>One/two-one cup strawberries</u>

<u>Dressing:</u>

- Pinch of sea salt
- One-two tablespoon. fresh lemon juice

- One-two tbsp. hemp seeds
- One-two tablespoon. olive oil
- Pinch of black pepper

What to do:

1. Assemble all items.
2. Blend entire what you need.

Serves- 2-3

Mouth watering Greek Cucumber Salad

Ingredients

- One/two clove garlic, minced
- Two-three teaspoons salt
- One/four-one tsp. paprika
- 1/4 tsp. paprika
- 2-4 cucumbers, sliced
- 1/4-1/2 tsp. white pepper
- Three-four tablespoon. lemon juice

- Four-five fresh green onions, diced
- One cup thick Greek Yogurt

Instructions

1. Assemble all items.
2. Slice cucumbers thinly, sprinkle with salt and blend.
3. Set away for 1 hour.
4. Mix garlic, lemon juice, water, paprika and white pepper, and set apart.
5. Squeeze liquid from cucumber pieces, few at a time and place slices in the bowl.
6. One thing remains to be done now.

7. Discard liquid. Now you should add lemon juice mixture, green onions and yogurt.
8. Blend and sprinkle additional paprika or may be dill over top.

Servings- Two-three

Insane Bacon Wrapped Chicken Livers

This recipe is quite simple and can be prepared under an hour.

What you need:

- 10-11 chicken livers
- Bacon slices as needed

Directions:

1. Assemble all items.
2. Wrap each chicken liver into one or two slices of bacon, securing it with toothpicks if needed.
3. Put the wrapped livers in a baking tray and cook in the preheated oven at 353F for 22 minutes or may be till golden brown.

4. Now serve the chicken livers warm.

Time: 45-48 minutes

Serves: 8-10

Out of the world Ceviche

I learned this recipe while watching TV. I made some tweaks to this recipe to suit my style.

Ingredients:

- Salt and pepper to taste
- Eight limes, juiced
- ¼ cup shredded parsley
- 4 tomatoes, chopped
- One half-two pounds seafood (scallops, red snapper, halibut, prawns)
- One-two sweet onion, finely chopped
- Two-three celery stalks, sliced

How to prepare:

1. Assemble all items.
2. Now wash the seafood well and chop it. Put it in a bowl.
3. Now you should add the lime juice and let the seafood soak up in the lime juice overnight.
4. The succeeding day, drain well and stir in the left ingredients.
5. Add salt and pepper if needed and then you can serve the ceviche fresh. Garnish with parsley.
6. Smell the aroma and serve.

Time: Eight½-nine hours

Servings: 4-7

Delicious Crab Parmesan Dip

What you need:

- Half cup grated Parmesan
- Half-one cup cream cheese
- ½-1 teaspoon dried oregano
- One-two can crab meat, drained
- One-two garlic clove, minced
- ½ cup mayonnaise

Method of preparation:

1. Assemble all the items at one place.
2. Combine entire ingredients in a small bowl and mix well.

3. Now serve the dip with vegetable stick or may be seed crackers.
4. Enjoy your day!!

Time: Twenty two minutes

Serves: Two-five

Beautiful Bacon Wrapped Shrimps

What you need:

- 24-25 bacon slices
- 24-25 fresh shrimps, peeled and deveined

Directions:

1. Assemble all items.
2. Wrap each shrimp within 1 slice of bacon and put them entirely on a baking tray.
3. Start cooking in the preheated oven at 350F for 10-17 minutes.
4. Now serve them warm or chilled
5. Enjoy your day!!

Time: 30-33 minutes

Serve: Six-seven

King sized Eggplant Chips
Ingredients:

- ¼ cup grated Parmesan
- Salt and pepper to taste
- 2-3 tablespoons olive oil
- 1-2 large eggplant
- One-two teaspoon Italian seasoning
- ¼ cup almond flour

How to prepare:

1. Assemble all items.
2. Now cut the eggplant within thin strips.
3. Please season eggplant slices with salt & pepper and place them in a baking tray lined with parchment paper.

4. One more thing remains to be done now.
5. Mix the almond flour with Italian seasoning and Parmesan. Then drop spoonfuls of mixture over every slice of eggplant. Drizzle with oil.
6. Cook in the preheated oven at 402F for 10-18 minutes and let them cool in the pan before serving.
7. Smell the aroma and then serve.

Time: 35-42 minutes

Serve: 2-3

Insane Garlic Baked Camembert

What you need:

- One pinch ground black pepper
- One-two tsp dried rosemary
- One-two medium size Camembert wheel
- Four-five garlic cloves, minced
- Half cup almond meal

Method of preparation:

1. Assemble all items.
2. Blend the garlic, rosemary, almond meal and black pepper in a bowl.

3. Put the cheese wheel in a baking tray and top with the almond mixture.
4. One thing remains to be done now.
5. Start cooking in the preheated oven at 352F for 32 minutes.
6. Now you can serve the cheese warm with seed crackers or may be veggie sticks.
7. Smell the aroma and serve.

Time: Forty two minutes

Serves: Four-five

Super Grilled Portobello Caprese

What you need:

- Salt and pepper to taste
- One-two garlic clove, sliced
- One half cups shredded mozzarella
- Three-four ripe tomatoes, diced
- 1-2 tbsp balsamic vinegar
- Four basil leaves, sliced
- 4-5 Portobello mushrooms

How to prepare:

1. Assemble all items.
2. Mix the tomatoes, garlic, basil and balsamic vinegar in a bowl. Now you should

combine salt and pepper to taste and then spoon the mixture within the 4 Portobello mushroom caps.

3. Top with shredded mozzarella.
4. Heat a grill pan or electric grill on medium.
5. One thing remains to be done now.
6. Put the mushrooms on the grill and cooking for 15-23 minutes until the cheese looks melted.
7. Now you can now you can serve the mushrooms warm.
8. Enjoy!!

Time: 40-43 minutes

Servings: 4-5

Powerful Pan Fried Asparagus

What you need:

- One-two pound asparagus, trimmed
- 2 garlic cloves, crushed
- ¼-1 cup olive oil
- Salt and pepper to taste

Instructions:

1. Assemble entire items at one place.
2. Heaten up the oil in a skillet and then you should add the garlic. Cook until golden brown then remove the garlic and discard it.
3. Put the asparagus within the hot oil and cook,

stirring often, for about twelve minutes.

4. Withdraw the asparagus on paper towels and top with salt and pepper to taste.
5. Serve the asparagus warm.
6. Enjoy!!

Time: 35-42 minutes

Serve: 2-3

Incredible Broccoli and Chicken whisk-Fry

What you need

- Four green onions, sliced
- One-two tablespoon oil
- One/two-one tsp xanthan gum (optional)
- One pound boneless chicken thighs, cut in bite-size pieces
- Four cloves garlic, minced
- 12-onethree ounces fresh broccoli florets
- Half-one teaspoons ground ginger

Sauce:

- 2-3 tbsps granular Splenda or equivalent liquid sweetener
- 1-2 tsp chili paste (sambal oelek)
- Two packets True Orange or other orange flavoring equal to approximately two tbsps orange juice
- 1/4 cup soy sauce
- Two-three tablespoons rice vinegar
- 1/2-1 teaspoon sesame oil

Method of preparation

1. Assemble all items.
2. Please heat the oil in a large or medium skillet or wok over medium or maybe high heat. Combine the

chicken; cook till the
chicken is done, stirring
occasionally,
approximately 6-8 minutes
or so

3. Now, please mix the sauce
   ingredients in small or
   medium bowl & please
   microwave the broccoli
   florets, in covered casserole
   or maybe the bag it came
   in, for two-four minutes or
   so on HIGH.
4. Please blend ginger &
   xanthan gum in a small
   bowl.
5. Smell the aroma and serve.
6. Makes three-five serve.

Stunning Low Carb Mushroom Chicken Dinner

What you need

- 1/2-1 pound mushrooms, sliced
- Salt
- 1/eight-one teaspoon pepper
- Salt and pepper, to taste

Sauce:

- 1/4 cup butter
- 6-7 chicken thighs
- One/four-1 tsp paprika
- One-two teaspoon soy sauce
- One/two-one teaspoon Dijon mustard

- Three/four cup heavy cream
- Dash paprika
- Pinch fresh parsley, chopped

Method of preparation

1. Assemble all items.
2. Season the chicken and put in a large baking pan. Bake at 427° for 45-48 minutes, until done. Approximately 22 minutes or so before chicken is done, and please melt the butter in a large or medium skillet.
3. Please sauté mushrooms until tender. Now, stir in the soy sauce & mustard,

then slowly stir in the
cream.

4. Please bring to a boil &
   then cook till the sauce has
   thickened.

5. Please season to taste and
   stir in parsley.

6. Now serve over the
   chicken.

7. Smell the aroma and serve.

8. Makes six-seven serve

Made in the USA
San Bernardino, CA
09 March 2020